HEALTHY EATING GUIDE

<u>Mastering the inner game of health</u>
<u>BY</u>
A.BASIT TIA

CONTENTS

INTRODUCTION

For some reason, one of the most difficult things for a human to do

is to eat properly. Whether this is due to our restricted access

to resources in all sectors, or whether we just have too many.

There are numerous reasons why people have so much access to unhealthy food.

Eating healthily is difficult.

Sure, humans can eat just about anything and survive. We

will manage to shift from one moment to the next and be able

to call ourselves healthy. Is it, however, healthy to live on a diet of

What about processed meals and sugary drinks? Simply because we are living.

This does not imply that we are in good health. And the more we age, the more our poor behaviors catch up with us.

It is immensely vital to create good eating habits early on in life, or at least, as early as possible to prevent any future issues from arising. You don't want to wake up one day and learn you've been deficient in nutrients for years, generating difficulties that are nearly impossible to correct. We must all take greater responsibility for what we put into our bodies since failing to do so can be exceedingly detrimental. Of course, when we are older and can reflect on our mistakes, hindsight is 20/20. We recognize that there were things we could and probably should have done but didn't because we were either unaware of the consequences or simply lazy. Simply knowing something does not obligate people to make a healthy-conscious lifestyle a reality. For the most part, we become more sensitive to how we treat our bodies and our health in general after being fully exposed to the misery that can ensue from bad health decisions. When we are unable to see the reality of our actions, the repercussions might look remote and difficult to relate to. We could even dismiss them. This may be a very debilitating situation to be in. Especially when you're already struggling with the consequences of bad eating habits and a lack of a nutritious diet.

Everyone deserves a chance to become the best version of themselves imaginable, but if we don't even acknowledge that unhealthy eating might throw us off track, even in the current moment, we'll be saying goodbye to the finest future conceivable. This book will help you understand the significance of eating well and how food affects our bodies and functioning. It might be tough to remain on track if we don't understand why our bodies react the way they do to food. However, there are several approaches to understanding why eating healthy meals is so essential, as well as how to embark on a healthy eating path. Let us not waste any more time. We should begin eating healthily as soon as possible.

CHAPTER 1: WHY SHOULD YOU EAT HEALTHY?

There are several reasons why eating healthy is vital. The majority of us are already aware of North America's rising obesity rate. This is especially true for the entire United States.

There is even a term for the way many Americans eat, which is known as the SAD diet.

The SAD (standard American diet) is a diet that is low in vegetables, rich in fat and sugar, and nutritionally insufficient.

Processed foods are included in the SAD diet. These are meals that are easy to get and cook, yet have long-term detrimental health repercussions. It is generally suggested that if you do not want to grow obese, you avoid eating such processed foods and instead focus on eating whole grains, fruits and vegetables, and meat that has not been treated with hormones or other chemicals that might wind up in your body and create issues.

Unfortunately, in North America, we have a lot of opportunities to slack off when it comes to meal preparation. We have so many options, and the amount of money required to purchase terrible food is significantly less than that required to purchase healthy food. It may appear unusual that buying organic costs more than buying foods that may eventually create health issues in the long term, but that is the rule of supply and demand.

Not only that, but processed foods are mass-produced and benefit enormously from their ease. That is why, in many respects, the obesity pandemic in North America comes as no surprise. Nutrition is not at the top of the list of corporations aiming to profit from people's inability to cook.

However, there are other reasons why eating healthily is crucial, as well as reasons to avoid processed foods and the conventional American diet. For example, if you don't want to be fat, you should read the rest of this book to learn how to change your nutrition and start living a better lifestyle. Another reason to eat healthily is that eating unhealthy foods and following a conventional American diet heavy in fat and sugar might put you at risk for illness. Diabetes is a condition that is often treated with healthy eating habits since it is caused by bad eating habits. Type II diabetes can be prevented and treated by maintaining healthy eating habits, but it can also be caused by poor eating habits. . If you wish to prevent these sorts of challenges and inconveniences, you should be mindful of your eating choices. Poor eating habits might also lead to other ailments. High blood pressure, as well as other chronic disorders, are frequent.

Osteoporosis can impact many people later in life because they did not make appropriate food choices when they were younger. You might end up with bad bone health, hypertension, or even heart issues. All of this may be quite taxing on your body and generate significant stress, which can be detrimental in the long run. Start making decisions today that will allow you to stay in their life for as long as possible if you want to show your family that you care. Poor health has an impact on everyone. It also affects others around you. It is pretty selfish for them to see you suffer as a result of the decisions you have made.

They are also in anguish. Now, try to make judgments that will benefit not only you but also your family in the long term. This book will show you how.

CHAPTER 2: UNDERSTANDING YOUR FOOD RELATIONSHIP

Everybody develops certain habits over time. We form habits in many aspects of our life. We form hygiene habits, eating habits, work habits, and a variety of other habits. However, they are typically completely unaware of our behaviors until they start to harm us. Even when we realize we are being negatively influenced by our behaviors, changing them can be quite tough. Because it is what I have, it is almost automatically something we do. We are conditioned to follow these behaviors, and breaking free requires a lot of willpower. When you recognize that your connection with food is based on the habits you've formed and can continue to shape and grow, altering your perspective becomes much easier. When you realize the importance of your future and make positive decisions about it, you are more likely to eat healthily and make decisions that will affect you and your future.

To be honest, many of us appear to be pessimistic about the future. We don't see enough reasons to change our ways because if we don't feel we have something nice to look forward to, it doesn't matter if we make good decisions or not. We don't see how we can shape our future to be beneficial to us. Most likely because we do not think we have any control over our life.

Don't be frightened if you recognize this sensation. It is a pretty frequent human experience. We are normally discouraged from taking control and exercising our power from a young age, and we may eventually cease feeling we have any influence over our lives because we are frequently told what to do by others.

That makes sense for youngsters. Children are not always aware of what is best for them. However, it may foster a powerless perspective, making it difficult to appreciate how the repercussions of our choices can genuinely begin to define who we are and how we show ourselves to the world. This is why it is critical to take genuine measures to better understand yourself and your food habits. When did you start doing it? How did you develop that habit? Why? What advantages does this behavior provide you? What are the negative consequences of this practice for you?

Ask yourself as many of these questions as you can so that you can properly comprehend how you are influencing your future with the food that you are eating. Are you creating a healthy and energized future, or are you's creating a future that is bleak and potentially full of negative health consequences?

Next, assess your level of self-discipline. Are you capable of exercising self-control over your choices? Or is this an area where you struggle? Discipline may be tough for everyone, and if you are having difficulty keeping disciplined, you should look into numerous methods that you can urge yourself to be a more disciplined person, both physically and psychologically. Only then will you have what it takes to go on a healthy eating path. Because, whether we like it or not, bad health choices are all around us. They are simple and addictive.

If we allow ourselves to be misled by these poor choices and do nothing to improve our behaviors, it makes little difference whether we eat healthily occasionally or not. The harmful consequences will continue to grip your body and surprise you when you least expect it.

In some ways, unhealthy eating is a self-destructive practice in which many of us engage. Self-destructive eating behaviors are harmful, whether they are caused by low self-esteem or simply because we are unhappy with our circumstances and have lost trust in the future. Before eating healthy to stay, you must first look at yourself and sincerely respect your life and future.

There are several methods to do this, and if feasible, you should seek the assistance of a mental health expert. They can sometimes help us recognize biases and unfavorable tendencies in our life that we are unaware of. Once things are acknowledged and accepted, it may be much simpler to overcome them and take the necessary measures to make great choices. There are several things you may do to change your thinking, whether you seek the help of a competent expert or not.

You will be willing to take the required efforts to achieve your goals as long as you feel you are deserving of a healthy body and a bright future.

It will be considerably more difficult if you don't like yourself. Understanding yourself, your habits, mental blockages, and discipline can help you along the way. Every day, we can work toward becoming our best selves, and eating healthily is a terrific place to start.

CHAPTER 3: DIET TRENDS CAN BE DANGEROUS

Diet trends abound in our culture today, and virtually all of them are fraught with risk. Unfortunately, most people who are thirsty for money sometimes fail to consider the long-term health repercussions of their products. What they are genuinely concerned with is generating money and producing something that will allow them to profit off the urgent need that many people have to lose weight quickly and easily.

If diet trends pique your attention, you'll have to accept one thing. Unfortunately, there is no good approach to losing weight rapidly, and simply that does not need any labor, proper food, or exercise. If you are fat or lack fitness and desire more mobility, losing weight is an excellent objective.

We have all been required to start making better lifestyle choices at some point, and that is something we can accomplish with food and good body activity rather than trusting businesses that seek to abuse us for profit.

Some food fads are extremely harmful and have serious long-term and short-term health implications. Many of them rely on procedures that deprive us and Robert's bodies of crucial nutrients. It can even dehydrate us. These eating habits are terrible. They prey on those who want to be healthy but don't know where to begin. They prey on people, generally women, who are cracking under the strains of artificial beauty standards, as well as on women who are persuaded that to be worthwhile, they must appear a specific way. You have worth whether you weigh 100 pounds or 700 pounds. Healthy eating, on the other hand, is one of the few genuine methods to jumpstart your metabolism and give your body the nutrition it requires to perform at its best. Not only that but there are health trends like the hCG diet that can mess with your body and hormones.

The irony of diet trends is that they frequently make it more difficult to lose weight in the future since you are using unhealthy and challenging methods of weight maintenance. If you want to be slim, don't put your faith in a medication advertised on TV. Begin by eliminating harmful sugary and processed meals and replacing them with nutritious whole-grain wheat and organic fruits and veggies that will not introduce chemicals into your body, making it even more difficult to lose weight and eventually messing up your body chemistry. It may appear appealing to be able to reduce weight rapidly without having to forsake the bad eating habits you have acquired over time, but this is not healthy. If you do not use caution when attempting to reduce weight, you will injure yourself and prime your body for future health concerns. Make certain that you are doing all in your ability to make decisions that you would like others to make for themselves.

Before you fall for the snake oil salesperson on TV, do your homework. Investigate these issues because you are worth doing things correctly, and you deserve a bright future that isn't muddled by the negative effects of a sales pitch that is just interested in your moncy rathcr than your health.

CHAPTER 4: FOOD PYRAMID

Most of us are familiar with the food pyramid. Growing up, the food pyramid was frequently used as a guideline to give us an idea of how much food and what type of food we should consume every day to maintain a healthy lifestyle.

Of fact, there is evidence to suggest that the food pyramid is flexible, but overall, observing the food pyramid will provide you with a rough notion of what is appropriate in a balanced and nutritious diet. While this might be contentious at times, it is still beneficial to have a baseline diet. Perhaps one that you design yourself. Many individuals would argue that eating as many grains as the food pyramid suggests is no longer regarded as the healthiest option.

In fact, with recent outbreaks of celiac disease, many individuals are promoting a no-grain diet as the healthiest option. Rather than using the food pyramid as a basic guideline for what is good to eat, think about your personal culinary experiences and go from there. A high grain diet may benefit some people., while others do not. Use your best judgment to the best of your ability in this situation so that you can take the best actions for your health.

The conventional food pyramid suggests the following:

• Rice, cereal, pasta, and bread can be consumed up to 11 times each day.

• You should eat three to five servings of vegetables and fruits each day, and two or three portions of eggs per day if you are not allergic or lactose intolerant. It is advised that you have two or three portions of meat and beans every day, as well as other foods such as nuts, fish, and chickcn.

•Unsurprisingly, sugar, fat, and oil are at the very top of the list. Because none of these things should be in excess. Rather, utilize them only as needed to maintain your healthiest lifestyle.

Once again, this is only a reference to the traditional food pyramid.

You may need to adapt this chart for yourself based on your own needs and dietary functions. However, if you do not have any special criteria, this is the food pyramid norm that may be used to your maximum advantage in developing a healthy lifestyle.

CHAPTER 5: HOW FOOD CAN BE

USED AS MEDICINE

Similarly to how not eating healthily may make you sick, eating nutritious meals can frequently treat illness and bring relief when you are suffering.

It can also be used as a prophylactic step against disease.

Ayurveda is a therapeutic system that has been practiced for thousands of years in India.

This traditional treatment method treats any condition simply by modifying your diet. Food has been the medication that has kept the people of India alive for millennia.

Many cures are just nutritious meals with anti-inflammatory characteristics and the capacity to nourish your body from the inside. Healthy eating habits have been shown to have an influence on anything from illness to cancer.

And that has never been more evident than with this ancient healing technique.

Of course, most current technology will dismiss these methods since they have not been scientifically explored, but much of it has been tried and true for thousands of years and will continue to influence the body. Whether you believe in the ancient healing art or not, diet can ultimately determine whether or not you are prone to sickness. If you eat healthily, your body will be stronger and better equipped to fight off disease and infection than if you were starved on the conventional American diet. Without the proper vitamins and minerals in your body, it can be difficult to fight off the negative effects of the disease. It can even cause disease at times. Certain types of uncooked foods might cause diseases and make you more susceptible to certain types of cancer if you consume them.

Although cancer is still being investigated and the scientific world does not fully understand it well enough to cure it, there are many examples of people who were able to live long and healthy lives, simply by altering the manner they require.

Healthy nutrition can assist to alleviate the symptoms of many tough and incurable conditions, such as multiple sclerosis. It will continue to do so as long as you ensure that everything you put into your body is nutritious and gives your organs and cells all of the fuel and resources they need to function properly. However, if you are intentionally destroying your body, it will be unable to fight as fiercely as it would if it were properly nourished. As a result, you must pay special attention to how you feed your body. If you do not make active and mindful eating choices, you may be setting yourself up for failure in ways that you will live to regret.

CHAPTER 6:THE ADVANTAGES OF EATING VEGETABLES

Vegetables are one of the world's most undervalued vegetables, especially in the conventional American diet. The importance of feeding the body with vitamins and minerals that veggies and vegetables alone can give is often underestimated. People are occasionally interested in veggies to improve their appearance, but when it comes to enhancing their health, they are less interested.

However, given that you are here and reading this book, it is reasonable to presume that you are ready and able to explore why eating veggies is vital. Here are some of the top reasons to include veggies in your diet regularly.

First and foremost, the body needs fiber to eliminate waste.

Without a way to collect and eliminate waste, it remains in the body and can contribute to weight gain and other potential complications.

Fiber is also essential for a variety of other reasons. It can help you prevent your blood cholesterol from rising and may even prevent or reduce your chances of developing heart disease.

Folic acid is also found in vegetables, and providing this substance to your body can stimulate the production of red blood cells. This can be extremely helpful in preventing anemia, and it is especially beneficial to women, who require this substance during pregnancy and menstruation. Vegetables are also naturally high in many vitamins, such as A and C, which aid in infection resistance and overall health. It can help you speed up the healing process and absorb iron, which is another way to help combat and prevent anemia. Vitamins are high in potassium, which is beneficial because it keeps the body from developing high blood pressure.

Vegetables have been shown to lower the risk of strokes and other cardiovascular complications. They can prevent the formation of kidney stones as well as the disintegration of bone matter. Consuming plenty of vegetables can help you manage type II diabetes and obesity. Not only that, but it can aid in your fight against cancer and cancer prevention. One of the most appealing aspects of eating vegetables is that they are low in fat and low in calories.

This means you can eat as many vegetables as you want without worrying about gaining too much weight.

Snacking on vegetables is a great way to help you control your hunger and maintain a healthy lifestyle.

Vegetables have so many wonderful qualities. Surprisingly, they are so scarce in the average American diet.

One of the best ways to help yourself avoid high fat and high sugar and high salt processed foods is by first walking around the perimeter of your grocery store.

Continue through the fresh produce section, making conscious choices to provide your body with healthy fresh vegetable options rather than skipping to the end and cheating by purchasing pasta and other processed foods that are low in genuinely nutritious vegetable content.

Choosing to nourish your body is the first step toward healthy eating, and few things are more nourishing than vegetables.

We often lose our taste for healthy foods as a result of unhealthy and poor eating habits developed early in life, or even self-imposed later in life, but it is simple to get back on track. Make room in your schedule for vegetables. They may take a little longer to prepare, but the benefits are well worth the effort.

CHAPTER 7: THE ADVANTAGES OF EATING FRUITS

People who follow the standard American diet do not eat enough fruit, which is unfortunate but common knowledge. What fruit they do consume is usually canned or sugar-laden.

The added sugar and fruit negate any health benefits that eating fruit in its natural state could provide the body. Excessive fruit consumption can lead to complications, especially if you have diabetes.

. Fruit contains a lot of natural sugars, and when you juice it, you gct a lot of sugar without much fiber, which can overload your body. One of the things that makes the fruit healthy is the fiber, which helps the body to lower heart disease and avoid constipation. Furthermore, fiber-rich foods such as fruits and vegetables are very beneficial for weight management because they help you feel full with fewer calories. Not only that, but the fruit is high in many vitamins and minerals, particularly vitamin C, which is abundant in citrus fruits. Vitamin C is a healing powerhouse, and if you're looking for something to help you keep your teeth and gums healthy, vitamin C-rich fruits will do the trick. Fruit can also help the body by preventing strokes and kidney stones. Fruits have numerous health benefits, including the prevention and treatment of diseases such as skin conditions and heart problems. Fruit is one of the healthiest ways to increase your energy and eliminate sugar cravings that you may experience when trying to eliminate unhealthy foods from your diet.

If you are willing to use the tremendous power of fruit,

you can have a healthy snack that satisfies your sweet tooth as long as you don't overdo it with your fruits, such as blending a bunch of them and consuming an absurd amount of sugar as a result. If you're curious about the health benefits of food, both fruits and vegetables have a natural tendency to make your skin glow and appear far more hydrated and nourished. Fruits and vegetables are high in antioxidants, vitamins, and minerals, which hydrate your body and keep your skin and appearance healthy.

It can help your hair grow softer and healthier, as well as keep your skin looking young. Fruit can even help you stop acne in its tracks by removing waste products from your body and hydrating your skin. Because of its high water content, fruit is excellent for helping the body stay hydrated, and you will quickly notice the benefits and that aspect.

Not only that, but the fruit is especially beneficial to digestion.

Because of the high fiber content, it aids in the binding of waste and aids the body in eliminating things that would otherwise cause problems.

As a result, fruits and vegetables can also help with weight loss.

Instead of allowing waste to be broken down and stored as fat, the body eliminates it before it can. Fruit is another excellent way to fight and prevent diseases, including cancer. Some fruits, such as apples, can help prevent asthma attacks. Others can significantly lower cholesterol levels.

Grapes, particularly red-skinned grapes, have been used in the treatment of cancer. They are also beneficial in the treatment of eye and kidney problems. Berries are especially beneficial if you have an infection. They contain a lot of antioxidants. Just make sure to eat fruits and vegetables that have not been treated with commercial pesticides, as these chemicals can absorb and complicate weight loss and cause issues in the body. You can even eat dry fruits to replace unhealthy and sugary snacks and provide your body with a sweet snack that packs a nutritional punch. Just be aware of the sugar levels in dried fruits, because when they are commercially sold, added sugars can turn what could be a healthy treat into something that will ultimately help you gain weight. Fruit, on the other hand, can help you lose weight if you eat it regularly and in a healthy manner. As long as you don't overeat sugary foods, the fibers and water content of fruit will help your body feel full and your cells and organs nourished. The fibers and water content will help you eliminate issues that contribute to obesity, and you will notice a significant improvement in your energy levels overall.

You can channel this energy into exercise and a healthier lifestyle. This is especially useful if you are replacing sugary junk foods with healthier fruit alternatives as you continue on your path to better health and well-being.

CHAPTER 8: THE HEALTHIEST MEAT TO EAT

Meat is widely considered to be one of the most important staple foods in an email, but you might be surprised to learn that some meats are healthier than others. We understand the distinction between red and white meats, of course. Red meat is more frequently associated with health problems and coronary artery disease, whereas white meat is considered leaner and healthier overall.

Some people may be surprised to learn that other factors

contribute to the unhealthy nature of meat. Issues such as what they are fed while the animals are still alive, as well as antibiotics and hormones, injected into them to make them grow faster or produce more milk, in the case of cows.

These hormones eventually make their way into the meat we eat and can cause problems in our bodies. If we are not mindful of the food choices we make, they can eventually contribute to poor health in the future, including but not limited to cancers and hormone changes that can be quite debilitating. However, if you are confident that your meat is coming from a healthy source that does not overfeed animals with steroids and antibiotics, you are already ahead of the game. If not, try to find local places where you can get meat that hasn't been tainted by dangerous industry standards.

Having said that, even among the healthy meat options,

some meats are healthier than others. Fish is one of the healthiest meats you can eat, especially if you're trying to lose weight. Fish is low in fat and high in nutrients. You must, however, be cautious about the source of your fish.

Some fish are raised in unsanitary conditions, while others may come from areas contaminated with mercury. This is why pregnant women should avoid eating fish or shellfish.

However, if you can find a healthy source of fish, it can be extremely beneficial to your body. Fish contains omega-3 fatty acids, which aid in brain function and memory. Overall, Omega threes are highly sought after, and the body requires them to function at their peak, particularly in intellectual matters. Another excellent option is chicken raised in a healthy environment. Chicken contains a lot of protein. It has the highest proof rating of any other meat. They are usually raised in good conditions or are fed foods that do not cause problems in the human body in the same way that a lot of beef does.

However, if you eat grass-fed beef from a reputable supplier, that can also be a great option. If you eat organic chicken, there is a lower chance that these animals were raised with dangerous carcinogens. Conventionally raised chickens are typically fed foods that accelerate their growth, which can result in serious health issues for both the chickens and the humans who consume them. They are also given an abundance of antidepressants and pain relievers, as well as arsenic and caffeine.

It is risky to consume a lot of conventionally grown meat, but if you can find a good supplier, you should.

Turkey is another excellent meat due to its high selenium content. This is advantageous to the body, particularly because it aids in the elimination of free radicals and other toxic substances. Again, you should try to get your meat from reputable sources because conventionally grown chicken and turkey are treated similarly and fed dangerous chemicals that unnaturally increase their rate of growth and eventually contaminate human bodies.

Eating meat in general can be very beneficial to the body, as long as it is not grown in hazardous or conventional ways. The chicken and turkey will be treated similarly and fed dangerous chemicals that will unnaturally accelerate their growth and eventually contaminate human bodies. Eating meat in general can be very beneficial to the body, as long as it is not grown in hazardous or conventional ways. The chemicals to which these animals are frequently exposed are extremely hazardous to both the animals and the humans who consume them. If you want to eat healthily and lose weight, you should avoid chemicals that may end up staying in your body and preventing weight loss.

Even if you don't want to lose weight, eating healthy means avoiding anything that could be harmful to your body, such as hormones and chemicals that disrupt our delicate systems. Fortunately, whether you prefer chicken, beef, or lamb, there are numerous sources of healthy meats.

There are options for getting healthy, ethically raised meat to satisfy any cravings you may have.

CHAPTER 9: THE PROCESSED FOODS ARE DANGEROUS FOR You

It should come as no surprise that processed foods are dangerous. What is surprising is that they are still allowed on the shelves, despite the havoc they cause in our bodies and minds. Eating unhealthy food is more than just a personal preference for some people.

People in poverty are sometimes forced to turn to processed foods because they are a cheap and easy way to feed large families on a limited budget. The problem is that these foods eventually cause medical problems that cost even more money than it would take to feed a large family with healthy, sustainable options. In the end, it appears that people with limited resources are suffering in either case.

Even if you don't have a family to feed, processed foods are simply unhealthy. Their high fat and sugar content contributes to their addictive nature. They frequently have boxed meals that include pasta and an excessive amount of sugar. Excess sugar is dangerous in general, but it is especially dangerous for people who are predisposed to type II diabetes. If you consume a lot of sugar, you will eventually overload your body, and you will not only become obese, but you will also develop health problems.

Sugar can hasten the progression of diabetes because it causes insulin resistance, which makes controlling blood sugar levels difficult, if not impossible.

If you eat foods like this frequently, such as for every meal or at least every day, there will be a negative effect consuming that much fat and sugar regularly can lead to not only well-known diabetes and obesity but also heart disease and even cancer. This is extremely dangerous, and processed foods should be avoided at all costs.

Another risk of eating processed foods is that they are not only addictive but also highly artificial. The majority of the ingredients in those foods are not beneficial to the body. Rather, they make us feel full while depriving our bodies of essential nutrients needed for healthy functioning. When we eat a diet that is bland and devoid of nutrients, we are ultimately dumbing ourselves down. We're not thinking, we're not moving well, and we're not performing to her full potential. All of these things are extremely harmful and can result in poor coordination and even depression.

On some level, we all understand that processed foods are not as healthy as the foods we should be eating regularly. Our bodies are aware of it, even if our minds are not. And we pay the price. We're worried about it.

Our bodies know when we eat unhealthy foods, whether we are addicted to them or not. And, whether consciously or unconsciously, we frequently punish ourselves. We are well aware that we are making a mistake. Even though we are currently processing it, we are upset and dissatisfied.

Artificial colorings, which are highly carcinogenic, are also abundant in processed foods. When we consume foods containing fixed coloring, we are essentially swallowing dye. Would you like to consume hair dye? Not at all. However, these are the chemicals found in your food. They remain in your body and do not leave. On the inside, they dye your organs.

They are extremely dangerous and can cause cancer.

They are also high in preservatives. Processed food lasts a long time on the shelf. Longer than is considered healthy and normal. A standard bottle of milk would not last for months on end.

It would curdle and go bad. The same goes for cheeses and other foods with long shelf lives that you can find on the shelves.

Companies must establish shelf lives because they can make more money if their food can stay on the shelf longer. They will do whatever it takes, no matter how harmful it is to the human body, to ensure that they make the most money possible.

Preservatives frequently contain harmful and unnatural chemicals, as well as excessive amounts of salt. Neither of these is good for the body. Because of the high salt content in these foods, processed foods can cause heart problems and hypertension. High blood pressure is common among people who live on processed foods, and obesity and heart attacks are among the leading causes of death in North America.

This has everything to do with the typical American diet. The unfortunate part is that even if you are aware that it is unhealthy, you continue to consume it. These processed foods are extremely addictive due to the chemicals and high sugar and fat content.

The body develops a craving for them, which can be almost as dangerous as drug addiction. Addiction to food that is neither nourishing nor healthy can have long-term effects on your health and development.

Another way that processed foods contribute to obesity is that we digest them much faster than foods high in healthy dietary fiber. If we digest these foods quickly and they do not fill us up because we are not getting the fiber that gives us a full feeling, we are not even using the same amount of energy to digest healthy foods. This means we eat more and digest less, resulting in rapid weight gain. When you eat processed foods, your body's calorie count rises dramatically. When you eat healthy, whole foods high in dietary fiber, you burn far more calories.

Unfortunately, this means that people who live and

thrive on a processed-food diet will gain weight whether they want to or not. And because they are not nourishing, they will not provide you with the same amount of energy.

They are likely to leave you tired, sluggish, and far too full because you eat far more of these unhealthy, sugar-filled foods without feeling content or satisfied. Our bodies do not properly metabolize processed foods. They quickly turn into fat. Furthermore, they are high in fat.

They are frequently high in hidden fat and sugars. Many of these processed meals contain vegetable oil as a primary ingredient, as well as high fructose corn syrup, which is a major contributor to weight gain.

If every processed food on the shelves contained high fructose corn syrup, which most do, it is no surprise that North America is experiencing the worst obesity epidemic in history.

Hydrogenated oils are extremely harmful because they do not degrade. They remain in your body and are absorbed by fat cells.

These oils make fat burning much more difficult. They are more difficult to eliminate, and this type of stubborn fat can quickly lead to obesity. The ingredients in processed foods lack the majority of the nutritional value that humans require to function at their best. Before we can truly thrive, we require the fibers, vitamins, and minerals found in real food.

If processed foods cannot be avoided entirely, they should be consumed in moderation. They are hazardous.

They can make us feel sluggish, irritable, and unsatisfied in general. When we go from a healthy diet to nothing but processed foods that are too sugary, too fatty, and unhealthy, our dispositions can shift from positive to negative. Our bodies are hungry. Providing that nutrition to your body is the simplest and most beneficial thing you can do for yourself. It can be difficult to adjust to new routines, such as relying on processed foods, and it can be very frustrating at times.

You'll have to spend a lot more time in the kitchen cooking and thinking about your health and meals. But, in the end, eating processed foods can kill you and cut you off from yourself. You are consuming toxins and avoiding foods that can act as antioxidants, giving your body a chance to rid itself of the waste that you are putting into it.

Processed foods are synonymous with junk foods. They are no exception. They appear to be healthier junk foods. They're snacks. Avoiding processed foods at all costs is the first and most effective step you can take to become and feel healthy. Don't be misled by packaging that claims these foods are healthy.

They are high in saturated fat, sugar, and salt, and low in anything that nourishes your body. Make every effort to break your dependency on processed foods. Eating healthy is simple and achievable if you put your mind to it. Remember the strategy of walking around the grocery store to get fresh produce and meat rather than walking through the aisles full of dangerous and alluring packaging that hides the dangers of the processed food within.

CHAPTER 10: MEAL PLANNING TIES IT ALL TOGETHER

One of the most important aspects of developing a healthy lifestyle is meal planning. When we are unable to see the future of our eating, it is all too easy to give in to the temptations of unhealthy foods to which we have become addicted. Especially if we have a habit of eating them instead of foods that nourish us.

Meal preparation is a time-consuming task. It can be intimidating, especially for someone who is affected by the organization. Don't worry if you're having trouble planning your meals. Whether you struggle with creativity in the kitchen or not, there are many ways to get started with fun and easy meal planning.

You can purchase a variety of meal planning kits. Many of them offer the option of ordering boxes full of fresh foods to cook with, as well as recipes. This can be extremely beneficial if you are unfamiliar with cooking, which is frequently the case. Especially when poor eating habits and a hectic work schedule make it appear difficult to make full, nourishing meals. Research is the first step in meal planning. If you want to get healthy, you need to consider your options.

The best place to begin is by researching recipes. Creating a binder full of healthy foods to try can be both entertaining and educational. It will open your eyes to several food options that you might have dismissed as too difficult for you to prepare, or it may teach you something you didn't know before.

Recipes can be very enlightening. Especially if you want to make discoveries. Cooking can be a difficult habit to develop, but once you do, you will be surprised at how much freedom you can find in preparing a meal for yourself that is both health-conscious and delicious. Look through recipe books and magazines for recipes that you want to try. Begin with what appears to be the most delicious and nourishing, and if you are a novice in the kitchen, you may also want to consider what appears to be the most simple. Next, keep your recipes organized in a simple, easy-to-navigate format. Meal planning will be made more difficult if you are overwhelmed by a lack of organization.

When starting a new habit, you want to make sure that everything is as simple as possible. Too much change at once can be taxing on your system, so always try to implement small, incremental changes.

Simple changes until they become a new habit.

Make sure they are easily accessible so that you can begin preparing your meal as soon as possible. If you use a binder, consider laminating the pages or using plastic sleeves so that they are not affected by water or other food contamination if you use it in the kitchen.

When organizing your recipes, put them in the order of breakfast meals, lunch meals, dinner meals, and snacks.

This will make it easier for you to find the right recipes once you start cooking. You could even organize your binder by day of the week if you want. and have your meals planned out for each day and printed in a binder.

There are numerous ways to organize your recipes. Do what intuitively makes the most sense to you. Don't force yourself to be a part of an organization that doesn't suit you. Instead, make sure you're doing what's best for you in your own life.

Make it a habit to seek out new recipes that stand out to you regularly to keep your creative juices flowing and your kitchen exciting. There are numerous recipes to try, and the more you try, the more interesting going on a healthy eating journey can be!

Following that, you should investigate Microsoft software such as Excel.

The office will assist you in organizing your meal

preparation. In Microsoft Excel,
There are numerous templates available to assist you.
Plan your meals by day, time of day, and week. This is possible.
be a tremendously useful resource!
There are also apps available if you do not want to use Excel.
could be downloaded on your phone, tablet, or another device
to assist you in making better use of your time and resources
You can also go the traditional route and purchase a notebook.
is specially designed for meal planning. This is significant.
step toward ensuring that your meals are well-organized and accessible.When embarking on a journey of healthy eating, having a meal plan is extremely beneficial. It takes time and patience to develop good habits, and you will inevitably slip somewhere

along the way. But that doesn't mean you have to remain on the ground!

It just means you'll have to get back up and try again because giving up is far easier than sticking to your plans.

Sticking to a theme can be beneficial when it comes to meal planning. Many people, for example, have specific themes, such as taco Tuesday or another day designated for a specific type of meal. If you believe it will help you stay on track, Feel free to replicate that type of meal preparation. It is done for a reason; it works and keeps things simple and streamlined.

It can be very inconvenient to be stuck doing a lot of planning and preparation every week or month, so if you want to keep things simple, this can be a good way to go. You could alternate between biweekly meals with a theme, such as a taco Tuesday one night and rice and vegetables Tuesday the next. There is no such thing as a bad way to plan your meals. What you must ensure is that you observe and follow through. Everything else becomes redundant and difficult without follow-through. Accountability is something that can truly help you succeed at meal planning. If you tell someone you know and care about that you are attempting to plan your meals, ask them if they would be willing to assist you in sticking to your routine.

They can assist you by inquiring about how things are going and whether or not you are on track. They may also choose to encourage and support you in your endeavors. They can be very rewarding for both of you, however, they choose to support you. If they are a positive and supportive person, it can be reassuring to know that you have people on your side who genuinely want you to succeed. Just make sure you're weeding out toxic people who bring you down by drawing attention to themselves or making you believe it will be difficult to achieve your goals. Sure, constructive feedback can be extremely beneficial, but it can also be toxic if you are not actively seeking it. Make sure you understand the difference between a toxic person who masquerades as supportive and a supportive person who genuinely wants you to succeed.

Another way to take accountability is through personal accountability. Personal accountability can be aided by journaling and self-affirmation. Talking to yourself about your goals, whether internally or aloud, can help you stay focused and ask yourself if you are accomplishing what you set out to do.

If you discover that you are not, rather than beating yourself up about it, consider your obstacles and move on as you discover them. The only way you will ever fail is if you never try.

Everything will eventually fall into place if you try because you are making an effort and making positive changes in your life.

Journaling is beneficial for a variety of reasons. They can assist you in writing down what you ate when you ate it, and how much you ate. This will give you a good idea of what you can expect from yourself realistically. Things you are dissatisfied with should be addressed and noted. But, rather than being angry at yourself for not becoming a trickle right away, remember that it is a process and that you must proceed slowly. Instead of implementing a complete change in routine and planning out every meal for the next month if you have never done it before, start slowly by easing into one or two meals a week and gradually adding in the rest as

you become more comfortable with the process.
Make it something that will not shock you. The most long-lasting change is gradual change. And journaling about your experiences will assist you in uncovering your innermost thoughts about the process as well as things that you may not have realized were holding you back. You will begin to notice patterns in your behavior and may be able to predict when and why you might be tempted to stray. It will be easier to avoid these trigger points in the future if you can identify them.
Meal planning can be a lot of fun and exciting. Even if you are not the type who enjoys that type of organization, it can be very rewarding to think about exactly what you are going to put in your body and to take the necessary steps to do so. Everyone deserves the opportunity to become the healthiest and most healthy version of themselves, and

with meal planning and a healthy dose of self-esteem, you will be well on your way to a healthy eating lifestyle.

CONCLUSION

Healthy eating can be difficult to start, especially if you were not able to develop healthy eating habits from a young age. It is, however, not impossible to become a more health-conscious and proactive individual.

Fortunately, every day that we wake up alive and breathing is a new opportunity to better ourselves and move forward in our lives. Being the best version of ourselves may seem daunting at first, but once you realize that every decision you make has an impact on your life, whether positive or negative, it becomes much easier to see the course of our actions before they come back to haunt us. Poor eating habits are decisions that will haunt us.

We will develop health problems later in life if we are not careful because we were not conscientious of what we put into our bodies when we were younger. The only way to achieve a healthy and happy body and mind is through proper nutrition and exercise. When we are cooped up in our homes all day, eating nothing but sugar and fat-laden processed foods and sitting around watching TV without moving, we become stir-crazy and restless. The typical American diet is hazardous and is costing people their lives. Make the necessary decisions to truly improve yourself and become the best possible version of yourself.

Make decisions that will make your family proud and keep you in their lives for many years.

When we do not take care of ourselves, we are being extremely selfish. People around us, whether we realize it or not, care deeply about the people we are and the value we bring to their lives. Everyone deserves the chance to shape their future and make positive changes that will benefit them for many years.

Healthy eating is only one of many ways to start bettering yourself and preparing your mind and body for the future.

If you want to be independent and active for as long as possible without spending thousands of dollars on medical bills and other expenses, you should start eating healthy sooner rather than later.

Otherwise, it will become a drain on your life, both financially and physically. You are now better prepared to take the first step toward a healthy lifestyle after reading this book and applying the information contained within it.

Planning your meals and becoming more aware of why making healthy food choices is important will improve your quality of life now and in the future. All you have to do is stick with it, and you will immediately notice the benefits of healthy eating! You've got this!

www.ingramcontent.com/pod-product-compliance
Lightning Source LLC
Chambersburg PA
CBHW061718130726
47996CB00006B/2392